Overcoming Bipolar Disorder

17 Ways to Manage Depression and

Multiple Moods without Going Crazy

Renae K. Elsworth

Contents

Bluesource And Friends

This book is brought to you by Bluesource And Friends, a happy book publishing company.

Our motto is **"Happiness Within Pages"**

We promise to deliver amazing value to readers with our books. We also appreciate honest book reviews from our readers.

Connect with us on our Facebook page www.facebook.com/bluesourceandfriends and stay tuned to our latest book promotions and free giveaways.

Don't forget to claim your FREE books!

Brain Teasers:

https://tinyurl.com/karenbrainteasers

Harry Potter Trivia:

https://tinyurl.com/wizardworldtrivia

Sherlock Puzzle Book (Volume 2)

https://tinyurl.com/Sherlockpuzzlebook2

Also check out our best seller book

https://tinyurl.com/lateralthinkingpuzzles

Introduction

Bipolar disorder is a condition that over 2% of America lives with. It is characterized by two distinct emotional phases: one of a depressive state, and one of a manic state, which can be expressed through a hypomanic or manic mood. The difference between hypomania and mania is essentially of degree. For some people, manic states are predicted by hypomanic states, but they both represent the manic side of the disorder. Opposite to mania is depression. Both the manic and the depressive episodes of bipolar disorder can vary in intensity.

The patient with the disorder experiences a shift between these two extremes. Some cycle between them within a few days, while others take months to complete the cycle. The reality for people suffering from bipolar disorder is a struggle to cope with these states while also addressing all of the standard responsibilities of life.

Often, symptoms plague people with the condition such as headaches, irritability, racing thoughts, low energy, and sleeplessness. These manifestations of the imbalance within the individual can easily affect their effectiveness in the workplace, their ability to recover from trauma, or their time management. Understanding how to cope with the manifestation of the disorder is crucial for the quality of life of those living with it.

To address this reality, many turn to medicine, and it is effective for them. This is a happy circumstance, and everything that works should be pursued. Many others feel their symptoms are exacerbated by pharmaceuticals, and there is a reason to listen to the body when it begins to feel disconnected or uncomfortable.

Both people who choose medicine, and those who choose to live without it, can heavily benefit from a holistic approach to the disorder. It may be accessed alongside or independent from therapy. The point is to address life completely and find balance so that harmony can be found within. Knowing how to balance through the extreme changes in their life is one of the most powerful tools a person with bipolar disorder can possess.

Below are 17 Ways to find your way to harmony with yourself, peace with the world around you, and understanding of your condition.

Chapter 1: Medications, the Implementation of them, and Managing Unwanted Effects

Psychologists understand bipolar disorder as a mood disorder that affects 2.6% of America. They believe it stems from a chemical imbalance, which is tied to genetic predisposition, or triggered by childhood trauma. The condition is characterized by distinct mood shifts.

To address this condition, several medicines have been made. If a person with bipolar disorder pursues traditional medicinal for treatment of their condition, then they will be placed on some level of medication.

The medications that the patient receives vary from case to case. Mood stabilizers are the most common prescription, but some patients also receive pills ranging from anti-psychotics to anxiety medication. Often, patients are put on a cocktail of pills.

For some patients, these pills will give them back their life. It will calm their mind, help them think clearly, and give them the motivation they need to take care of themselves. For other patients, an attempt to solve one issue will only worsen another. It depends on how it affects you.

What's most important is that the condition is addressed. The difficulties that come with pursuing medication don't excuse living with an untreated disorder. Taking care of yourself is your responsibility.

Likewise, it is your responsibility to do what you feel comfortable with. If you've tried pills and they make you feel better, then you have no reason to stop. If you've gotten on pills and find it hard to create, hard to enjoy things, or you feel like you're sleeping through life, then consider pursuing another option.

It depends on how your body reacts to it. Some people smoke into their hundreds, while others are allergic to water. What's good for you and what's poisonous for you can only be understood through experience.

The doctor will have a lot of good information for you. It's good to build up a relationship with a therapist, because they have seen hundreds of people with similar conditions to the one that you have.

This means that they are a great resource for identifying strategies you can implement in your life, and how to avoid falling into the common problems that affect people in similar circumstances.

What you need to keep in mind is that healing is your responsibility. You can lead a horse to water, but you can't make him drink. No matter how much assistance you receive from other people, it will ultimately be your responsibility to manifest the effects in your life.

You are responsible for the maintenance of your mental health. If you do not commit to the strategies that are made available to you, then they will not work. You need to want to get better. If you are being prescribed pills, take them or else you're wasting money and time. There's no point in pursuing something that you don't think will work.

Talk therapy can also be pursued independent from medicine, and there are more obvious benefits from it. Since the beginning of human history, we have gone to elders for understanding. In the modern era, we make this into an occupation, but it fulfills the same function, where someone who has had experience in the world can prepare someone else for what they have to face.

Follow your gut, and be whoever you are comfortable being. Medication is an incredible tool for many people in coping with their condition. If it is a positive contribution in yours, then commit to it. If it's questionable, then address the other circumstances in your life, such as your diet and your social standing.

Chapter 2: The Cycle of Energy and Finding Alignment

Bipolar people exude energy. Whether they do it positively or negatively depends on where they are on their cycle, but still, their ability to channel it is powerful. They extend well into the extremes of either side of their emotional spectrum throughout their life, chasing fever dreams, and not leaving their bed for entire days. Without proper self-care, bipolar people are prone to utter imbalance.

The modern understanding of mental illness only came around recently. Before that, we didn't see mental instability as different from the norm; different societies had different interpretations. From the Greeks to the Native Americans, there were spiritually awakened seers. This hints at understanding people have had for longer than recorded history; a sense for tension and the flow of energy. Many of the symptoms of bipolar disorder match up with the descriptions of these people.

Overcoming Bipolar Disorder

If you can understand the emotional sensitivity as a spiritual sensitivity, it will become obvious why balance and moderation are crucial for the bipolar person. Their heightened experience of moods and the world around them leaves them to being utterly overrun with their own feelings and experience. This isn't because they are dramatic; it's because they're more in tune with emotions that are too large for them to understand.

To make this gift more comprehensible to people in general, bipolar people must moderate their experience and translate it into something that can be largely accepted. This doesn't mean that bipolar people must learn to become inauthentic, but that they must learn to become presentable.

We are social animals who depend on our abilities to communicate within groups. If we are not able to reach out to our fellow person, then we will fail. As the world becomes more and more urbanized, socialization becomes more and more of a factor in a healthy life, despite the growing trend of isolation. Bipolar people will benefit heavily from maintaining a connection to others, because people will help them understand what the healthy limits of emotions are.

An even lifestyle will also help balance the energies of the bipolar person. Most of them are drawn to excitement and adventure, but those aren't what they need. Chasing after their fantasies only encourage their energies to grow. Instead, they must commit to their lifestyle and let themselves grow to expect consistency in their circadian rhythm, maintain regular eating habits, and experience healthy conversational standards. The more normal a life they are able to maintain, the more even their emotional flow will be.

Different people want different things from life, however. Not everyone who drinks needs to go to Alcoholics Anonymous. Some people will require more excitement in their life, while some will require more stability. The point isn't to get the athlete to stop risking their bodily health. The point is for you to be able to depend on yourself.

When you have your own trust, everything will become easier to manage. The anxiety that you felt before will be met with your own competence. Finding balance in life doesn't give you the same adrenaline as staying up for a week, but it also means you'll never have to feel your heart falling out through feet.

For most bipolar people, it's much better to commit to a stable life than to cling to the sensation of excitement that mania leaves you with. You're not a good friend to yourself when you're chasing after dreams that you can't reach. You feel how you treat yourself. Remember that, tend to your needs, and find the center within yourself. Once you carry everything you need within, there will be no longing for anything outside of yourself. You will be secure.

Chapter 3: Deep Breathing and Presence

To start working on anything, you must first address it. If you want to better yourself, you need to be able to find yourself. This means understanding that you are a soul within your body, and that your body is your moment-to-moment reality. You need to be able to feel yourself, to understand what it is that you are.

Breathing is an excellent place to start, as it is one of the few things we need to be in the process of every moment of our lives. Find a position you're comfortable in; one from which you will not move. This is important. You'll need to stay like this for at least twenty minutes. Once you've found it, find where your eyes rest. If there's a neutral place in the room, then place them there. If you want to close your eyes, then do so; whatever helps you find peace.

Take a deep breath, filling your lungs as fully as you can. Hold it for a moment, feel it inside yourself, then let it go. Count the inhale and the exhale. Think the words "1" and "2" on the alternation. So, for example, "1" on the inhale and "2" on the exhale. You can also count

"1" on the exhale and "2" on the inhale. You can also replace the words "1" and "2" with any other single syllables, so you could use "peace" and "love" if you wanted to. Find words that you can channel without much thought.

Count your breath as you look at nothing. Think about nothing. When thoughts come into your mind, release them. Either bubble them away or burn them without engaging them. Become neutral; find your way back into the animal state. Breathe in the air around you, and then exhale.

As you find yourself, let go of your ego. Don't let your presumptions come to you. Let your body speak. Your muscles will come alive and your blood will flow. Life will occur even as you don't consider it. We're not as monolithic in our existence as we assume. Enter a state where your existence is the only process that you are undergoing.

When you do this, you are essentially restarting the system of energy that you carry around. By embracing your animal reality, you are causing a hard reset. Your energy will be allowed to figure itself out again, figuring out the proper pathways that it needs to take for you to be able to manifest it.

Like running hot water down a clogged drain, deep breathing meditation clears the channels of communication within our soul.

This will help the bipolar person regulate their emotions, because there will be more bandwidth for those emotions to flow through, so they won't be restricted by narrow elbows.

All muscles need to rest, and so does the soul. This is why meditation benefits humans, especially those suffering from mood disorders, so much. If you run on your legs for months, then they will wear down and become less functional. The same applies to your emotional capabilities. Disengage from the situations that you find yourself in, and take the time in your life to simply be you. The attention that you give yourself is one of the foundations of stability.

This practice should be repeated. Some religions require you to pray several times daily, so there is enough time in the day for you to meditate. Also, the more time that you set aside for your health, the more that you will communicate to yourself that you are worthy of your own resources.

Chapter 4: Managing Your Chakras

The entirety of the universe is the expression of energy. Matter is energy in solid form. The chakras are the points where your energy is manifested into reality; they make up your existence as it continues every moment.

Each chakra is responsible for different emotions and bodily functions. Your issues with your stomach may point to an imbalance with your Solar Plexus chakra. To balance that, you may need to start committing to the truth and living your life authentically.

Many bodily issues can be traced by to chakra imbalances. In Western Medicine, we aim to fix the symptoms, but in alternative medicines, they consider the entire body. Eastern traditions have traced mental and physical issues back to energetic imbalances for centuries.

This knowledge is worth considering, because it is powerful if you can manifest it within yourself. Spiritual energy can be an incredibly healing and balancing influence in your life. If you can grow a healthy relationship with it, then you will benefit from the security it offers.

Reiki practitioners are a great resource in managing your energy. After you experience trauma, or if you were raised under challenging conditions, then you will carry those burdens in your energy. It will haunt you after it happens, because it lives on in your memory. Reiki can cleanse you of this burden, and help you learn to let go.

Once you can cleanse yourself, you can repair your relationships with your chakras. Your journey with each of your chakras will be unique. Different chakras require different things to open, although they all work in harmony. Studying color and the sonic arts will help you learn how to manifest your energy.

Respecting this knowledge will help it be effective. If you believe in your energy, you will be able to feel it flow. Visualization is an important part of the practice; you have to trust your imagination. Doing so will help your mastery over yourself, because you will experience how you navigate the metaphysical.

As you work with the esoteric, you will learn about yourself and about how others perceive the world around them. This knowledge is incredibly valuable for learning balance and how to express to the world around you. The deeper that you understand energy and the chakras, the more you will understand about how energy is manifested, and why people act the way they do. Once you have that knowledge, then you can find alignment with it.

Chapter 5: Engaging with the World around You

As social animals, we learn from the standards that are held by the people around us. It's hard to guess what these standards are without experience, so everyone must gain experience in the judgment of others. The lesson that bipolar people need to learn is how to express emotions appropriately.

By learning the standards of others, bipolar people can pick up on what healthy emotional regulation is. This can help them learn how to better regulate their own emotions and how to lead a more stable lifestyle. Ultimately, bipolar people are normal people; they just need to know how to find balance with themselves and their condition.

Through learning how to be a part of a community, and how to be a good influence on other people, we learn what healthy expression is. This is crucial, because it takes the same delicacy to tend to yourself that it does to tend to others. Through being socialized with other people, we understand how they deserve to be treated.

What this aims to illustrate is that emotional abuse is not normal. People don't want to be dragged from one height to another depth within moments; nor do they want to run through the extremes for months and ruminate on all of their wildest thoughts. It is impolite to project this emotional energy out onto other people, and the public does not respond positively to it.

With this example, the bipolar person can learn that they don't want to be treated like that either. They will learn to respect their moods and give them space, rather than allowing the extremes that they feel encroaching on them to run their psyche. Just like you have to wait your turn to speak in conversation, the bipolar person will be able to push their emotions into their proper place.

This is because you respect that emotions take time to unfold. A good novel is not filled with a whirlwind of feelings and desperate plots; it is made of well-tuned threads that keep the pieces together. Understanding this, you will understand that emotions need time to prove that they're worth your attention.

Our whims should not dominate our lives. That is being our own bully, dragging ourselves along to whatever we want to see. Our intuition should have to prove itself. We deserve an explanation for what we are being asked to do.

By insisting on this standard within their self, the bipolar person can enforce moderation in their life through self-trust and self-respect. This is a healthy frame of mind.

Being in the right conditions will promote this attitude within the bipolar person, which is why it's recommended for them to have a rich social life. Having a healthy community will have the greatest effect, and whether it's filial or geological is unimportant. As long as they can contribute to something with a standard they can learn from with good intentions, they'll be in the right place. It will either heal them over time, or they will struggle too much and lose the opportunity.

If rejection from a community occurs, it isn't an issue. It will provide you with the experience and wisdom that you need to succeed in the future. Take note of what behaviors made it so that you were no longer welcomed there, then be sensitive about expressing them in the future. See if there is a way you can meet people in the middle.

If you can internalize healthy lessons from your experiences, you will be a blessing to whatever community you become a part of. The more you are able to be a healthy influence on others and promote healing, the more healing will take place within you.

Chapter 6: Going to a Doctor

The modern doctor is a modern convention. It's good for certain things, like vaccinations and fixing broken bones. When it comes to the mechanics of human beings, it excels, but past that our conventional doctors leave something to be desired.

The pharmaceutical industry has had too large of an influence on the medical world to be ignored. Many doctors prescribe for a profit, because they have incentives from certain companies to promote certain pills. Most people who are prescribed one pill require several others, leading to cocktails of five pills or more for some patients. If it works for you, then that is a good thing. Use whatever has come into your life with positive energy.

For those who want more options, they exist. Several affordable alternative health options are available across America. There are people who offer acupuncture, there are psychics, there are people who truly practice yoga, and there are people with experience in healing the body.

Overcoming Bipolar Disorder

People who have bipolar disorder have a lot of energy flowing through them, and many struggles to balance that. Instead of restricting those energies through chemical caps, Reiki and acupuncture aim to cleanse the body to allow the chakras to flow evenly. Several people prefer the experience of working with the body instead of against it.

There are also several herbs that can be beneficial for bipolar disorder. Seeking out people with knowledge about what herbs might benefit you could be as effective as any other methods. Some people only require certain supplements; magnesium has changed a lot of peoples' lives.

It is important that you have guidance on your journey with bipolar disorder. Trust the traditions that you choose, but trust someone. Some people benefit from Chinese medicine, while others need mood stabilizers. Everyone is different, and everyone is comfortable with different things. The best thing is to follow your gut and experience the paths that you consider worthwhile.

Listen to other people with the condition and see what worked for them. Many bipolar people benefit from joining a spiritual practice, so see if there is a community of healthy people with a spirituality you can jive with. If you can, consider opening up to spiritual healing as another option.

Wisdom exists in everyone, and it can be expressed anywhere. If we could contain wisdom, then we wouldn't need freedom. All of the best ideas could be hoarded. Instead, we all have our contributions to make. This means your intuition is as good as anybody else's. You get to try to see what works just like the rest of us do, so be brave enough to figure it out for yourself.

This doesn't mean that you should do it all yourself. Find people you can trust and listen to their guidance. Everyone needs support from outside of themselves. Find healers, but find healing through the channels that you trust, and that you have had good experiences with. Just because something is official, it doesn't mean that you have to trust it.

The more that you can engage your healer with trust, the more their work will be effective. The human body is better at getting better when it wants to. By working through things you believe in, you will commit to the changes and strategies that you want to become a part of your life.

When you own your healing, then it will work. No one else can do it for you; they can only provide the tools to do so. Regardless of where you get your resources from, you have to learn how to use what you have been given. Due to this, make sure to pursue support from places that you feel comfortable supporting back.

Chapter 7: Engaging with Holistic Knowledge

There are several ways for you to begin your journey with holistic knowledge. The simplest way is by grocery shopping. Start cooking all of your own meals only using plants and vegetables. Make your own flours, but try to avoid bread. Many bipolar people are negatively influenced by caffeine, gluten, sugar, and anxiety medication. All of these things promote imbalance within your energy, and so it will spread imbalance into your psyche. By eating a clean diet, and deriving your energy from food instead of chemical supplements, you will feel much cleaner and fresher. It will leave you with more energy to address life.

Other than diet, there are many forms of holistic healing. In most major cities there are herbal shops and crystal shops. Those establishments usually carry literature on holistic knowledge and hold classes on them. Getting involved in those communities is a great way to become introduced into holistic knowledge.

There are also practitioners of healing, such as psychics and acupuncturist, which can provide alternative medications. You may need to take on certain rituals into your life, such as burning certain herbs to cleanse your energy, or to obtain certain crystals. Harmony with external reality is not to be underrated.

What's great about holistic knowledge, is that you can engage it at your own rate. Find what interests and you and test it out. If it works, then make it part of your routine, and internalize the ceremony. If it doesn't, then move on. You don't stand to lose anything by experimenting with alternative healing, and it's an interesting story if it doesn't work out.

The experience of the healers is real, though. Some people accredit them for doing away with pain, cleaning them of trauma, and healing digestive issues. If you can trust people, then there's something to this community.

Don't throw money at it, but find affordable services you can try. Get your palm read and see if anything you learned from it comes up in your life. Go for a Reiki session. There's no promise that it'll work, but medication doesn't work for everybody. The more methods that you try, the better chance you'll have at finding balance within your life.

This community is also welcoming of bipolar people. To them, it is not something that needs to get fixed, but an expression of your energies. The way to address imbalance is to bring that expression into healthy fruition.

Chapter 8: Engaging with Your Body

Systems do not exist because we name and observe them, and nature is perfectly happy to exist without our influence. Your body is very complex. It is an independent system of organisms that collaborate to power a large being. Within the complexities of their relationship with each other, your consciousness is contained.

This is why finding yourself is so important in the process of healing. You are not your thoughts; you are yourself. You don't communicate to yourself with words; you communicate with yourself through feeling and sensation. It's a primal engagement between self and body.

Your body will carry your energy and your habits within itself. It will ache from what you rely on too much and be weak where you forget to exercise. This is true for muscles, and it is true for your emotional fiber. If you understand your feelings, then you will find many useful things you can do to address them.

By listening to yourself, you find a wealth of information. You will start to notice how certain people and environments make you feel. You will be able to see how your hobbies affect your mood. If you can acclimate to healthier eating, then you will also see the effect of food. All of these things will teach you what you need in your life.

Your body has standards that you didn't imagine. It responds better to different diets, and different schedules. A regular sleeping habit can change your life, especially for people with mood disorders. The better that you take care of your body the better your psyche will hold together. When you respect yourself, you notice that respect.

Yoga is a great practice for finding alignment with your body. Most people have postural problems, and practicing yoga will help them learn about them. It will also give them examples of how to build the muscles they need to correct their posture.

Posture isn't an aesthetic thing; it's a health thing. If you don't hold your weight evenly, then different parts of your body are forced either to work harder or to work under conditions they're not familiar with. It puts unnecessary stresses on your body that can lead to serious issues.

This is why it's important to correct how you hold yourself. You should drink water, eat foods that make you feel good, which aren't negatively affecting your health, and find ways to exercise. The more that your body is able to exercise its existence, the more motivated it will be to be a part of it.

A large part of depression is not wanting to be alive. When you're not invested in life, and when your body doesn't feel well, why would you want to be? Addressing bodily issue evens out the struggle to stay motivated in life. Achieving happiness is something many people have difficulty doing, and things like chronic discomfort will only get in the way. Treat yourself to a healthy body, it will make everything less dramatic.

Chapter 9: Engaging Knowledge

You are not the only one with this condition. There are thousands of others, dead and alive, who have been affected by it. Due to this, there are many resources that you can pursue to access information about the disorder.

Several writers, historical figures, and people in your community have had experience with bipolar disorder. It's not news to the world; it's something that's been around for centuries. As you reach out to the world, you will find there is a lot you can learn to help manage your condition.

There are many people who thrive with bipolar disorder. Influencers ranging from Kanye West to Yung Lean are affected by it, and they are vibrant parts of their cultures. Difficulties may arise in their lives, but they still pursue meaning, and are able to express themselves through their mediums.

Overcoming Bipolar Disorder

Many other people have made it their life's work to spread information about this condition. There are several resources worth your consideration, but it depends on what you are attracted to. Some of the communities are heavily medically influenced, presenting information in a measured environment, and there are other communities that focus on experiential and emotional approaches.

Video testimonies are a great resource for seeing what kind of information clicks with you. By seeing how people talk about the condition, you can feel out how your own thoughts align. Most people have their own feelings about the condition, but once you find someone who shares your attitude, follow their references. See where they're getting their information.

By working with leads that you are emotionally attracted to, you will find information you'll naturally retain. The most important part of planning to overcome bipolar disorder is to have a strategy. The cycle will hit again, and you should understand how you need to prepare.

This is why finding people you respect is important. Once you find a way of thinking about the disorder that you feel is valid, you can internalize the strategies of that community. Some believe in deep breathing and crystal meditation, while others believe in medication.

Overcoming Bipolar Disorder

There are hundreds of ways that people have successfully coped with this condition. Some people use meditation, some use religion, and others use community engagement. Studying the strategies that others implement is like comparing recipes with a fellow chef. You don't need to cheat, but there's always inspiration you can take.

Be creative with your approach. If you have bipolar disorder, it's yours as much as it is anybody else's. There is the medical definition of it, but you can manifest your soul however you chose. Figure out what the feelings mean to you and how to express them. Make use of what you don't understand. See what others do, and join in the attempts to translate your experience into something. Everyone contributes to our understanding.

Chapter 10: Group Therapy

No one with Bipolar Disorder is alone. This is a human condition that thousands of normal people have. By socializing with other people who are coping with the condition, you can normalize living with it and not feel like you have to figure things out for yourself.

Unstructured environments are not the best for group therapy. Bipolar people don't need to confess to their previous addictions; they need to have a good example of emotional regulation set for them. Due to this, they benefit more from structured group environments while learning how to cope.

Sports are an example of a good environment for development, because they place the objective off of emotions and onto collaboration. The social element is focused, so the rules become more obviously understood.

When group therapy can work with a similar philosophy, it is especially effective. Putting the focus on self-expression in a group doesn't help, because it's ruminating on symptoms. By engaging in positive group therapy with direction, you are embracing a proactive approach, which encourages positive behavior in the participants.

The way that you're socialized is very important. It affects your opinions, the way that you speak, the way that you act, and many other things in your life. Group therapy is an attempt at socializing you again, into a standard that leaves you with more self-respect and genuine care for yourself.

Group therapy can also be especially effective as a guide for how to treat other people if you struggle to set boundaries. For those who struggle with aggression and inappropriate expression, group therapy can be a slowed down guide for how social interactions are supposed to go.

These symptoms can be incredibly well addressed with group therapy, because many bipolar people simply haven't been exposed to a healthy standard. It's not that they don't want to act better; it's that they don't know how to manage their condition in a way that is societally appropriate.

By displaying tools that work to do exactly that, manage life in a socially functioning way, group therapy can provide bipolar people with the examples and practice they need to hold themselves to a healthy mindset. It doesn't work for everyone, but it is especially effective for people who weren't exposed to many people in their childhood, and those who were exposed to toxic people.

Chapter 11: Managing Thoughts

Racing thoughts are not quick; they're repetitive thoughts that you can't break out of, like a tick. Several bipolar people suffer from this symptom without truly understanding it. They think that's how the brain works, that you get focused on something and it doesn't leave your head. This is actually an example of obsessive thinking, with racing thoughts being a pattern you can't escape.

These thoughts are usually negative in nature. In depressive moods, these thoughts can manifest through internal insults. They may attack the bipolar person's appearance, their sexuality, their ability to socialize, their place within the economic system, or anything else that can be judged.

Without knowing what these are, people may think it's insecurity or a lack of confidence, but it's not. It's a toxic thought pattern. This is why it's of paramount importance to stop the cycle. Deep breathing is a good first step in the process.

Overcoming Bipolar Disorder

After you are able to find presence and let go of all your pent-up energy, build with positivity. Build with self-affirmation everywhere you used to have doubt and hate. Commit to stable thoughts of support and belief. By building yourself up, the negative thoughts won't be able to take you anywhere; you will be able to stand your ground.

If you can't manage to become neutral, then force yourself to be positive over your pathological negativity. As you force yourself into the direction of healing, you will gradually override your predisposition for hostility. If you follow every negative thought with a more powerful, positive thought, you will start to become wired toward positivity. This is a savage way to break out of your thoughts, but sometimes they follow you too far for you to be polite.

Mania has its own manifestations of racing thoughts. These vary widely from person to person, because mania can manifest through symptoms ranging from euphoria to irritability. What makes a manic state is a rise in energy—a low-grade rise in the hypomanic state, and then a potent one into the manic state.

In the manic state, obsession can become an issue. Romantic obsession is especially dangerous and needs to be limited. If you can't control your thoughts about someone who doesn't know you or want to communicate with you, then create distance between the two of you—the less they are a part of your life, the less you will think about them.

Work obsession is another common manifestation, along with purchasing mania. All of these must be controlled for a good life. Create space for yourself and commit to yourself as a person, not an idea. Engage with deep breathing, eat foods that are good for you, and take time to invest in the activities that you want to be present for. The more that you can focus on the life around, you the less energy will be available for you to obsess.

While in a mixed state, racing thoughts can be truly dangerous. This is when the issue of suicide is to be the most considered. Through the drop in mood and the rise in energy, a bipolar person in a mixed state can easily fall into a cycle of lurid, self-hating thoughts. These thoughts can eventually lead to visualizations and auditory encouragements of suicide.

If you suffer from these thoughts, you must learn to control them. Meditation cannot be recommended enough. When these emotions come in and out of your life without your control, there is no chance for you to gain stability.

Find someone you can be with when your thoughts get bad. Don't vocalize them, but try to find another frame of mind. Talk if you have to, but try not to give any place in your life to toxic thoughts. Attempt to live past them, to return to what makes you feel good.

Chapter 12: Managing Anxiety

Fear is a good instinct. It's correct for your adrenaline to start pumping, and for your hair to stand on end, when you are in the presence of a predator. This response allows you to react to the danger more adequately.

When you respond like this consistently while there's no danger present, you're likely to have an anxiety disorder. Bipolar people tend to have a comorbid anxiety problem. Racing thoughts can worsen this issue.

Different people have different triggers for their anxiety. Some people are only affected by social situations; others can't be around certain sounds without extreme discomfort. Fear is a learned reaction, so your fears are dependent on your experience thus far.

The best way to train against this, and to address racing thoughts, is to commit to proving it incorrect. If you are afraid of driving at night, take a road trip across the country in the summer. Face your fears in a way that allows you to prove they are manageable.

If you're afraid of confrontation, you should learn to be assertive. The more experience that you have with people, the less the anxiety will flare, because as you condition yourself to the situations you are afraid of, the fear response will fade.

Anxiety is a bodily response that's subconsciously trained. It's not because of the thoughts you think, or the way that you live your life; it's because of experiences you internalized. To move past it, you must teach yourself in the same way you learned: through experience.

By seeking out positive experiences and affirming yourself with them, your body will grow to expect that, instead of the negativity your anxiety stems from. Our mental health is an accumulative object, so the more time you spend setting these habit for yourself, the more secure they will become.

It's important to know what to do in the moment too, and it's almost always what you need to commit to—if you can or disengage if you can't. Sometimes a drop of courage is enough for you to navigate a situation, while other times there's too much stimulation for you to keep your head straight.

Recognizing the difference will require you to have an honest view of yourself. You need to know how many resources you have at your disposal and how to manage them. If you have enough strength to go through a situation, then try to commit to it. The stronger you can be, the less fear will dominate you.

However, there is no reason to expose yourself to a losing situation. If you know that a circumstance will lead you to stutter uncontrollably, cause you to be irritable, or cause an otherwise negative effect, then avoid it. Turning away from triggers isn't running from your issues; it's using your energy wisely. There will be similar situations that you will be able. There is always more opportunity to learn.

When you choose these situations correctly, then your anxiety won't hold you back. Everybody is limited by something, so having your own considerations to take into account is nothing unique. You're playing the same game as everybody else, trying to make the best that you can out of a flawed being.

Don't fear anxiety, but know that it's largely a concern about nothing. You are okay and you will be okay. Your life will improve as you take care of it. Once you're an adult, you can gain control over your life. Inherit the responsibility for yourself and do well.

Chapter 13: Opening Up to Loved Ones

Therapy should carry the largest burden when it comes to balancing your feelings. You can pursue that therapy in any way you feel comfortable, but it is important that you deal with problems yourself. This is because everyone is responsible for their own health. You will never be able to outsource that to other people. If you attempt to do, so it won't end up well.

Once you are able to bear your burden, then you can be vulnerable with the loved ones around you. Do not expect them to address the majority of your emotional reality, but be honest with what you experience. Feel comfortable expressing your history and your interests. Be present with those who are close to you.

When you develop your close relationships with honesty and understanding of your condition, you will find your way through intimacy. It's difficult to do so when the disorder is untreated, because there's such an abundance of energy in the life of a bipolar person. Once balance is found, then the true value will be added to your life.

Many bipolar people feel like they are in some way more flawed than the average human being; that they are lesser for their condition. This leads them to self-isolate and disconnect from their relationships. It is important to fight this feeling, to push it away and embrace a positive reality.

There are people in your life now who care about you, and there will be more people who care about you. There is always an opportunity for you to build upon profound relationships in your life. Approach them with an understanding that you want to be healthy, but don't be afraid.

It won't be hard to be around those who are important to you after you have adapted to social standards. Social standards exist so that people can be around each other easily; so that everyone can interact while feeling comfortable and safe.

Having a mellow and measured way of responding to the world will go a far way in interacting with those around you. By tempering your response to the world, you will demand less from those interacting with you. Your peace will spread to those around you, and they will feel grounded while exposed to you.

Overcoming Bipolar Disorder

The more grounded you can be in your relationships, the more they will flourish. Time is what nurtures all things, so if you maintain healthy boundaries, then your relationships will deepen and remain healthy.

Family is provides excellent environment when they are supportive. Make sure they support the measures that you take to better yourself, but also trust and engage with them. They're the people who you come from, so they will often be there for you. Stability is important, not only in recovery from mood swings, but in the prevention of them.

Romantic relationships can also provide a lot of support in your life. If you can find a healthy level of consideration that really helps you achieve balance, it's not too much to try to maintain a healthy environment. Ask for what helps you. Habits aren't a bad thing to have, and historically some of them were called ceremonies.

Respect others and respect yourself. You will find that way you have many resources to improve your life, and that you are able to add value to the relationships that already exist in your life. A healthy life is one in which you give and take. Learn balance in that and all will follow.

Chapter 14: Emergency Plan

Sometimes life reaches a point where there so much drama and energy flying around, that a person with bipolar disorder can feel overwhelmed. These situations can lead to incredibly stressful situations, as they would for anyone else. It's good to recognize when these triggers happen and how to seek out help during them.

While you don't want to use others to process your feelings for you, if you're experiencing an especially terrible low or high, calling a loved one is a good idea. If you can be with them physically, that is also a solid option. The social pressures from being around people we respect can calm our anxieties. Support from the people in your life will do more than you think.

There are also methods that you can do alone. Find a park that you enjoy staying around and map it out. There are hills that you'll find charming and plants you'll want to learn about. Invest your time into places like these, and they will be a refuge for you in the difficult moments.

Spending time taking care of yourself can also be as simple as going out for a quiet coffee, or a massage. Take time to repair. When you feel too much pressure, you're probably too stressed, so relax and get ready to take on new projects.

If you feel especially at risk, try to find people to be around immediately. If you are experiencing racing thoughts about suicide, contact a professional. At a certain point, there are crises that aren't your responsibility to solve. Once you start having a seizure, it's time to give someone else the task of figuring out what needs to happen.

It's okay to be at a loss with life. If you can accept that, you will be able to deal with everything. All stress passes. When you're strong enough to deal with your problems, you really have none, but only things to get done.

Accepting difficulties makes them manageable. Stop running from a crisis and you won't be too tired for it. Be patient and handle everything that you can. Wait to see if there are steps for dealing with the things you don't understand how to cope with. You can probably come up with something, or you will figure it out while you're not thinking about it. If you keep hope—then everything is fine.

Finding calm is the important path through any episode. Identify what the problem is, and assess what level of risk you have. If you need to make calls because your life is at risk, then it's better to make them. If you can forgive yourself, settle down, and adapt back to being okay, do so.

Stress will not be useful in this situation. The less panic you allow to spread, the safer you will be. Use deep breathing and other meditations. Give yourself space and understanding. Everything will be okay if you wait; there will be a new day, new seasons. Life never stays the same.

Chapter 15: Creative Expression

The creative fields have benefitted from bipolar people since they started. Bipolar people make for wonderfully passionate contributors in every field across the human interests. Many of those bipolar artists find art to be an excellent valve for their energy to have.

Art is a realm in which there are no limits. While it's inappropriate to test out all your thoughts on other people, it's okay to do so while practicing an art. You can find true liberation by engaging in realities and perspectives that don't affect our own reality. There are no negative consequences that come from being confused in art. Admitting that you have more to learn is the best way to become experienced in the craft.

All of the arts have had a history with bipolar people. One of the most famous examples is Van Gogh. It's hard to diagnose dead people, but through his biography, the habits are pretty faithfully described. He goes through periods of utter inertia, and then is the most active and kind person in the village, right before turning into the vilest person his brother ever met. Still, despite the struggles of his life, his contributions to the vocabulary of art continue to define the modern art world.

Of course, you shouldn't aim to live a life like Van Gogh's. The point is that even the most talented people share this condition, not that we should emulate their lives. The best artists often leave little to envy the lives they lead. Just don't feel like there's any reason your expressions will be limited by bipolar. Geniuses work with it too.

A stable relationship with art can give you an alternative language in which to interface with the world around you. If Van Gogh did not have painting, then he would have been lost. Meaning can be found through the arts. It shouldn't be the only thing that you define yourself, but it can get some people through struggles.

All arts have emotional capabilities. Even writing, perhaps the most rational of the arts, has great emotional depths. Any of the classic plays can prove the capacity of that medium for emotion. Feel free to explore with any medium that speaks to you.

If you've never had any training in the arts, and aren't capable of breaking into them, then you can find opportunities to learn. Thousands of people want to share their interest in art, and many of them are passionate about introducing others to what gives their lives so much meaning.

This can happen through acquaintances, classes, school, or anything else where you can regularly interact with someone about an art form. Sometimes it doesn't even need to be the same person, as long as you keep talking about art with people in general. As you gain experience, you will find the space to practice.

Each art form has its own vocabulary. Spoken language is limited, because it's meant to be understood. Rarely, if ever, are we making sounds to be interpreted for their own expression. There is an abstract meaning behind the sounds that are directly important to their expression.

This is not true in typography, or in drip-painting. As you learn a medium, you will learn a language unrestrained by the needs of explanation. Emotions don't need to have the limits of rationality within them; the more truthfully you can express the emotions you have within yourself, especially the ineffable ones, the greater the value of your work will be in revealing truths about the human condition.

Flexibility is a virtue. If you become well versed in many things, then you won't be at a loss for how to handle reality. Maturity in expression will always be valued.

Chapter 16: Community Significance - Substance Free Lifestyles

Your body wants to live a healthy and successful lifestyle. It wants to be in balance with itself and to be strong. If you respect and know how to communicate with it, it will bring health into your life.

Many people address bipolar disorder without allowing any substances in their life, herbal, medicinal, or otherwise. These people also tend to have a tremendous amount of social support in their lives. There are many ways to heal from the world, and if you have enough healing energy, then you don't need every tool made to address the situation.

This approach is interesting, because they prove the healing mechanisms are within the bipolar person. If they want to practice true self-mastery, then they can achieve a relationship with life where they control the disorder. Being prone to feeling intense emotion does not mean that you have to express intense emotion.

Overcoming Bipolar Disorder

Once you can channel even the most extreme feelings through yourself with moderation and grace, there is not much danger in continuing the lifestyle that you have chosen. The most important thing for a bipolar person is to find an acceptable balance that allows them to function within the world. Once they have achieved this, they have found the center.

Most mental disorders, from drug addiction to PTSD, can be healed incredibly well through healthy socialization. Humans are their influences, so by being exposed to good influences, people learn better habits. If you're part of a good community, the lessons they surround you with will become imprinted on you.

Due to this, having a strong relationship with a community addresses the majority of some bipolar peoples' issues, while being a great coping tool for others. For those who are socially sensitive, it can provide them with the boundaries and the hope that they need to face life. In their case, being connected to the world around them is all they need for balance. Expression is enough to let go of the excess energy.

For others, learning how to manifest the energy within themselves will relieve great pressure from their inner systems. Energy is not supposed to stay stagnant; it is supposed to flow and be free. By not knowing where to place energy, bipolar people will suffer from it building up within them.

Having the ability to talk about yourself and your experiences is a fundamental skill. It's crucial in becoming better, and the more skilled you are at expression, the better you will be able to heal. Not only will you be able to join communities, but you will be able to express yourself to healers authentically and accurately.

By building up your social sense, you will be able to better access the resources that exist for people to cope with life. No one is expected to live without difficulty; don't feel bad when you need others to help you through yours. All you need to do to deserve it, is be available when the people who help you need assistance.

By being balanced externally, the bipolar person can set healthy standards. That standard can then be reproduced, internally, and socially, to balance out their relationships in general.

The more experience they have with healthy interaction, the easier it will be for them to take part in it. By being part of communities that value them, bipolar people can prove their value, and even when they suffer from their lows, their value will not be forgotten. People care about people, and they remember one another.

Chapter 17: Alternative Medicines - Food, Herbs, Non-Addictive Substances

The advantage that alternative methods have over pharmaceuticals is that they're non-addictive. When you try them, you won't build a literal dependency on them that can trigger an episodic shift. Your chemistry will be safe.

They are medicines as much as they are lifestyles. You can't take a pill for your chakra; you must clean it and maintain it. You must live well to feel better; that's the philosophy. Holistic healing is a journey into learning what it means to experience life as a human.

A controversial conversation can be had on substances such as cannabis. For many people with bipolar disorder, this herb is utter poison, as it throws them into paranoid panic fits. For them, it should be avoided as much as possible. For others, it dampens their mania while helping them through their depression. These people can embrace it as a tool.

Other herbs are useful, such as sage, different teas, kava, ginger, and more. All things grow for a reason, and many of them can be consumed. Your reaction to them will be unique to your body, so experiment with what the world has to offer, and how it affects you.

You are made of what you consume. Drinking water is a highly underrated cure to many issues. While you're well hydrated, your energy can flow better, and you can recover from whatever you need to. It also helps deal with headaches and fatigue, and sometimes relieving those burdens can reveal a lot of resources that weren't available before.

Good food contributes to a good life. If you consume nutrient-dense things and exercise, your body will appreciate it. It's not about looking better or gaining confidence; it's just easier to exist when you treat your body well.

By having a focus on foods your body can use, your diet is working for you rather than draining energy from useless matter. The less work you force your body to engage in, the more energy will be left over. As you introduce stress into your life, you reduce quality. Your work and your life will become worse.

Take a broader perspective on your life and internalize the knowledge that works for you. Address your life for the whole that it is; engage with yourself spiritually, emotionally, and patiently. Listen to what makes sense for you.

Conclusion

After this conversation on bipolar disorder, I hope you have found yourself able to cope with the manifestations of it in your life, or that you can share this knowledge with someone you know who has the condition. If any of this was useful to you, please spread what you learned, as knowledge about self-care may be the piece that someone needs to get a hold of their lives.

The condition affects many gifted people, the artists, the powerful, the humble, and everybody else. There is no shame in having it, and the self should be embraced through all features. Nothing means that you don't have a right to love and promote yourself.

Please take care to be patient with yourself and those around you. Figuring out life is difficult, especially when you have a condition that affects your emotional state. Take the time and resources required to reassess your needs, and find your way to supply a lifestyle for yourself that keeps you happy and healthy.

Finally, if this book was useful to you, please become vocal. The more activity that we can have within this community, the more information can be spread and understood. It's essential that this knowledge is social, not studied, so if you could mention this work or review it on Amazon, that would promote this knowledge becoming more public. Thank you for your time. I hope your journey goes well.

Renae K. Elsworth

Overcoming Bipolar Disorder

Connect with us on our Facebook page
www.facebook.com/bluesourceandfriends and stay tuned to our
latest book promotions and free giveaways.